AN INTRODUCTION TO COMPUTERS IN GENERAL PRACTICE

THE FRIENDLY WAY TO LEARN WHAT YOU NEED TO KNOW

by

Dawn Allison Dip, MAMS
Computer Manager, The Limes Medical Centre,
Theydon Bois, Essex.

PUBLISHING
INITIATIVES
BOOKS

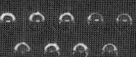
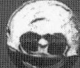

ABOUT THE AUTHOR

Dawn Allison was recruited as a programmer at The Bank of England in 1978. During her time there she was trained in various programming techniques and languages, and gradually expanded her role into systems analysis. She was also involved in investigating the possibilities of microcomputers, newly arrived from the US in the early 80s. In 1991, she joined The Limes Medical Centre where she is now Computer Manager, responsible for all aspects of computer use in the practice.

ACKNOWLEDGEMENTS

A big "THANK YOU" to:

The doctors and practice manager for backing my further education endeavours.

My fellow computer operators for 'holding the fort' while I attended college.

John Dawe, my excellent tutor, who encouraged all my efforts to achieve my AMSPAR goal.

Especially to Alex, my 'other half', who spent evenings alone but has supported my efforts throughout this project.

First Published 1997

Printed by Biddles Ltd of Guildford and Kings Lynn.

ISBN 1 873839 39 1

Further copies of *An Introduction to Computers in General Practice* can be obtained from Pi Books, a division of Publishing Initiatives (Europe) Ltd. This publication reflects the view and experience of the author, and not necessarily those of Publishing Initiatives (Europe) Ltd.

CONTENTS

3

SECTION FIVE

SECTION SIX

4

SECTION SEVEN

SECTION EIGHT

SECTION NINE

SECTION TEN

SECTION ELEVEN

SECTION TWELVE

SECTION THIRTEEN

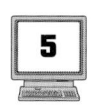

PREFACE

I would like to present you with my computer experience to date and, in so doing, give you an insight into my reasons for writing this guide.

While working at The Bank of England, I was trained in logical and methodical programming techniques, which taught me to write mainframe computer programs for specific office tasks and to identify and isolate problem areas within programs and other software. I was also shown techniques to test my programs thoroughly and confirm with the eventual system users that this was exactly what they wanted. Finally I provided the users with training and documentation.

My role gradually expanded to systems analysis, for which greater skills and awareness of office protocols were required. I learnt to utilise flow diagrams to show users how their systems would operate in their office environment.

Whilst carrying out all of these tasks, I used various programming languages, dependent upon which type of system I was designing for - mainframes, minicomputers (minis) or microcomputers (micros) - now known as personal computers (PCs).

Most of my present knowledge about PCs was gained from my experience in this area, and from useful hints and tips from colleagues who already had some experience with these systems.

I find that nearly every day in my current role at The Limes Medical Centre, I draw on my experience gained over these 12 years. Most of all I find that my knowledge is useful to many people in many ways, and something I may take for granted is worth its weight in gold to others working in GP surgeries.

My studies on the AMSPAR Practice Managers Diploma course and questions raised there, have brought me to the point where I believe that this guide would be very useful as a reference in many GP surgeries.

This guide should help you choose and use your computer wisely and safely.

It is not necessarily meant to be read from cover to cover; I have endeavoured to provide succinct sections with helpful headings to allow you to discover just the item you wish to find out about. However, some areas do overlap.

I have tried, also, to cover most topics that people generally ask about, including areas such as concepts, terminology, buying, maintenance, expansion or just plain "what do I do?".

I could never hope to include all subjects, as computing is a fast-moving growth area. However, I trust some of the mystique is explained and you will find something of use for yourself or others.

D. Allison

Dawn Allison Dip, MAMS

7

GLOSSARY OF COMPUTING TERMS

Those words printed in bold can also be found in the glossary with their own definition.

BACKUP	A daily procedure which copies information to external media (i.e. **tape cartridge** or **disks**) for safe storage elsewhere, in case of loss or corruption.
BUG	A fault in a **program,** manifested when it does not carry out what was expected.
BYTE	One unit of **data** or **memory,** consisting of eight bits.
COMMUNICATIONS	The linking of one computer to another to exchange information, e.g. Health Authority Links.
COMPATIBILITY	The ability of different manufacturers' equipment to work together successfully.
COMPUTER	A mechanical or electrical machine that can manipulate numerical data or other stored items of information.
CONSUMABLES	The materials that are used up daily by any computer system, e.g. paper.
CPU	The Central Processing Unit or microprocessor. See **processor.**
CRASH or HEAD-CRASH	An abrupt halt to computer processing, brought about by an error in a program, a corruption of **memory** or power fluctuations.

CURSOR	The point on screen at which the system waits for **data** entry from a user. Usually a block or underscore, static or blinking.
DATA	Anything that a computer can manipulate, such as numbers, text, diagrams.
DATABASE	A method for organising lists of information, such as patient names and addresses.
DISK	A form of media storage. See also **diskette** and **hard disk.**
DISKETTE	A form of media upon which **data** is stored externally to the system, usually 5¼" or 3½". For small amounts of data.
DOT-MATRIX	A type of **printer** that fires fine needles onto an inked ribbon in arrangements that form characters and symbols.
DOWNLOAD	A procedure which copies information from one computer system to another, via any type of **media** or connection.
DUMB TERMINAL	A screen that gets all its information from the main computer with no ability to run other programs.
FONT	A specific design of characters, also known as a typeface, used in **word processors,** for example Times Roman.
FORMAT	The way data is stored in **tracks** and **sectors** on a disk.
FORMATTING	The action of marking out magnetically the tracks and sectors onto a disk.
GIGABYTE	1,024 **megabytes**.
GRAPHICS	Diagrams or pictures displayed on screen, now usually in colour for PCs.

HARD DISK	The medium upon which data is stored inside your computer. Divided into **tracks** and **sectors**.
HARDWARE	The physical components of your system, such as the **processor**, screen, keyboard or **printer.**
HELPLINE	A direct contact point with your system supplier when a problem occurs or advice is needed.
ICON	A graphic representation of an action that can be selected by pointing with a mouse. Used in Windows packages.
INTELLIGENT TERMINAL	A screen that can carry out instructions from the main computer using special **software**, but has memory of its own to run other programs.
KILOBYTE (Kbyte or K)	= 1,024 **bytes** (2 to the power 10).
LANGUAGE	The special format instructions that are passed to the computer.
LAPTOP	See **portable PC.**
MACRO or HOT KEY	A series of keystrokes that you would normally press individually to enter **data**, which can be put together and executed using one special key.
MAILMERGE	A way of collating a large number of addresses with a standard letter.
MAINFRAME	The largest type of computer.
MEDIA	Any materials upon which data is stored, e.g. **diskettes.** Also any materials upon which data is printed, e.g. paper. See **consumables.**

MEGABYTE (Mbyte)	= 1,048,576 **bytes** or 1,024 **kilobytes.**
MEMORY	The method by which a computer stores data in an organised fashion. Usually by electrical or magnetic means.
MICROCOMPUTER	A computer designed to be as compact and as easy to use as possible. (Synonymous with **personal computer (PC)**.
MINICOMPUTER	An intermediate size of computer, between **mainframe** and **microcomputer.**
MODEM	Short for modulator/demodulator. This is the 'box' that converts computer signals into telephone signals and *vice versa*. This allows computers to communicate along telephone lines.
MOUSE	A small device that partially replaces the use of keyboard depressions by pointing to images on screen to select an action. Mainly used for the operation of PC packages.
MS-DOS	A proprietary name - Microsoft Disk Operating System. This is a type of **program** that controls the components of your computer system and allocates sufficient space to the **software** you wish to run on it.
MULTIPLEXOR	This is a 'box' that allows several pieces of equipment at a remote site to communicate with the main **processor** at the same time along one telephone line.
PACKAGE	A set of **programs** that are usually sold together, arranged so that information can be passed between them. An example would be Microsoft Works which contains a **spreadsheet**, **word processor**, **database**, charts and **communications**.

PERIPHERAL	A device that is connected to the main computer, e.g. **printer.**
PERSONAL COMPUTER (PC)	A computer designed to be used by one person, originally for home use.
PORTABLE PC	A computer designed to be carried around. Sometimes called a laptop or 'luggable'!
PRINTER	A mechanical device attached to a computer that prints text.
PROCESSOR	The central processing unit (**CPU**) that carries out all arithmetic and logical operations, the nub of all programs.
PROGRAM	A set of instructions to a computer that are carried out in order.
PROGRAMMER	One who writes a **program** for a computer.
RAM	Random Access Memory - a special area of **memory** used by your system software and packages.
SECTOR	The smallest amount of data (256K) that is read at any one time by the computer. It is usually 10% of a **track**.
SCREEN	A device for displaying information from the main **processor** to the user for identification and action.
SLAVE PRINTER	A printer that is attached directly to a **terminal** for its sole use.
SOFTWARE	Sets of grouped instructions or programs for the computer.
SPREADSHEET	A particular type of program that allows entry, display and printing of **data** in rows and columns (tabular format).

SYSTEM	The computer and all of its attachments.
SYSTEMS ANALYSIS	Understanding how a task is performed in order to write a **program** to achieve the same goal.
TAPE CARTRIDGE	A form of media upon which **data** is stored outside the system. For a large quantity of data.
TERMINAL	A screen and keyboard unit displaying information from the **processor**.
TRACK	This is an area on a disk where data is stored in a circular arrangement, not physically discernible. These are subdivided into **sectors**.
UPS	Uninterruptible Power Supply. Used to level out variations of power and prevent damage to **data** in the event of power loss.
USER	The person who sits at a screen entering or using the **data** displayed.
VDU	Visual display unit - see **screen**.
VIRUS	A particular type of **bug** that is transmitted between **programs** without detection and renders the system partly or totally inoperable.
WINDOW	This is a section of your screen that can be used independently. It gives the ability to 'juggle' different tasks that might be required to run at the same time, whilst allowing the user access to each one on the screen.
WORD PROCESSOR	A type of program that allows easy manipulation of any text, with different **fonts** and styles. Can be used to produce standard letters and mailing lists.

1

DECIDING ON A NEW COMPUTER SYSTEM

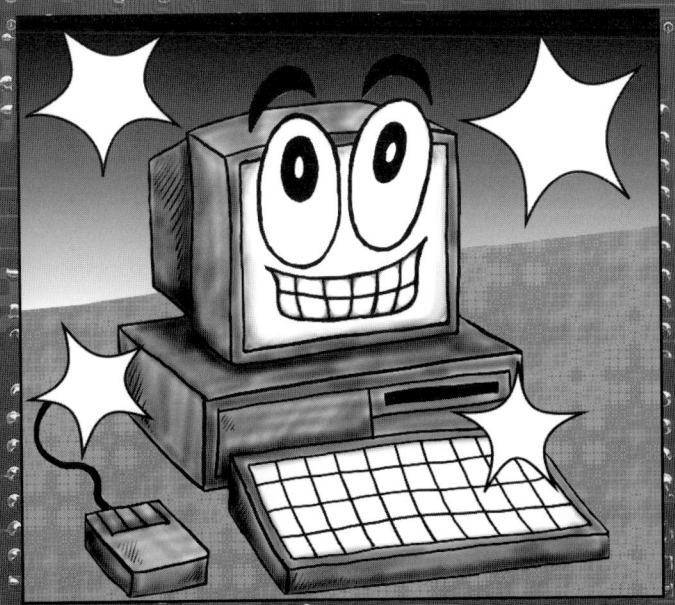

DECIDING ON A
NEW COMPUTER SYSTEM

Do you know exactly what you want a new computer system to do?

This is the most important question to ask, not only of yourself, but of all the practice staff. Everyone will have slightly different views about what a terminal sitting on their desk could achieve for them. Pooling together all these ideas would help to draw up a short checklist to be taken to any future system demonstrations.

Every practice is run in a different way and a new computer system should complement the way you work, although some clerical changes may be required. Decide on the main areas you want computerised first. These would normally be the age/sex register, medical records, prescriptions and appointments, perhaps followed closely by word processing. Identify any ancillary staff who have expertise or interest in these areas to aid you in finding the best system for your particular needs.

Once you are ready to look at different options, approach your Health Authority, which usually has a computer department and staff willing to help. They can give you a list of the latest computer system suppliers that have gained 'accreditation'.

ACCREDITATION

The Information Management Group (IMG) of the NHS Executive has set guidelines for all suppliers of hardware and software within the general practice and hospital environments. Those that have reached these standards are given NHS approval via 'accreditation'. Make sure your Health Authority supplies you with a current list, as companies and their status are changing regularly.

DEMONSTRATIONS

This is the most important part of buying a computer system. It helps to clarify what you want from a computer system and how the system will work in your practice.

Below are some guidelines on how to go about organising demonstrations, what to look for in a good computer system and what questions to ask the suppliers.

Go to demonstrations armed with a checklist of your requirements. Always make a note of your first impressions of the system - its use of menus, colour, helpful layouts, on-screen information boxes, etc. These are the things that make using the system more enjoyable.

However, do not forget the practical aspects for comparison with other systems.

The following is a checklist for demonstrations at other surgeries:

DEMONSTRATION CHECKLIST

❑ *The number of GPs in the partnership.*

❑ *The number of patient records held on the system.*

❑ *The number of terminals linked to the system.*

❑ *The number of printers.*

❑ *Any branch surgery links?*

❑ *How long the system has been in use.*

❑ *Any problems encountered on installation.*

❑ *Any problems encountered with hardware.*

- *Any problems encountered with software support.*

- *Any problems in changing the system (whether from manual or previous computer systems).*

- *Do GPs and nurses have one each and use it during consultation?*

- *Are they using any links to third parties, e.g. path labs, Health Authority?*

- *Is there anything they particularly like about their system?*

- *Anything they particularly dislike about it?*

- *How long does backup take?*

These are all things you need to find out about the general running of the systems at demonstrations. This will help you with a comparison of systems at a later stage and will help to clarify whether this system would benefit your surgery.

Immediately after each demonstration, write a brief description of the system using the checklist points and any other items of interest that you jotted down at the time. It is often impossible to remember which system did what after a number of visits. Try to use the same format for each description.

Having seen a number of systems, shortlist those that seem to suit your needs best. Then invite the supplier to give you an in-house demonstration of the system. Make sure that you get a representative from each group of staff to attend these demos, as they may highlight potential problem areas that might not have occurred to you.

The demonstrator should be able to give you a thorough look at the system and answer any questions you may have. They will probably use a portable PC which they bring with them. Don't get excited if it is in colour - you may not get this on your final system. Ask the demonstrator about this.

COMPANY CHECKLIST

Now is your chance to ask some crucial questions about the company itself:

- ❏ *How long has it been going?*
- ❏ *What training do they provide?*
- ❏ *What telephone support is given?*
- ❏ *What response times are guaranteed on software and hardware problems?*
- ❏ *Whether support is usually carried out via a modem link to your system? (If this is the case, you will probably need a separate telephone line.)*
- ❏ *How many systems they have supplied to date?*
- ❏ *Are there any local surgeries that have this system? (This is so that you can have a chat with them.)*
- ❏ *Will you be able to add on extra terminals, and link to branches, the Health Authority and path lab?*
- ❏ *Is this supplied as standard and therefore included in any quote you might receive, or is it an 'optional extra'?*
- ❏ *Will you be able to upgrade to a processor with greater capacity at a later date?*

This is also the time to firm up your requirements, such as the number of terminals and printers that you will need. Use your own judgement, but listen to the demonstrators, as they are often able to suggest modifications that might suit you. They will then

20

go back to their office and send you a quote for the system you have specified. Remember that when you ask for a quote you are not committing yourself to that company and are free to shop around.

Have a short meeting among yourselves after the demonstrator has left, while the details are still fresh in your minds. Decide whether you all agree that this is a suitable system - get everyone's impressions now.

After a few demos you will probably know which one to choose. Most of the systems you will have seen are very similar and it's down to common sense and personal choice at the end of the day. If you are still unsure, have another chat with the surgery that uses this system; this would probably clear your doubts.

OTHER FEATURES TO LOOK FOR

Software
Most accredited systems now supply the following within their software:

- *Patient register*

- *Appointment system*

- *Clinical recording*

- *Consultation recording*

- *Search facility*

- *Reporting facility*

- *Mailmerge (standard letters with patient details)*

- *Patient printouts*

- *Audit trail*

- *Fundholding*

Ensure that the system you choose has these main facilities. Some systems also incorporate other features, such as:

- *Mentor - a clinical diagnosis system based on the MUMPS database.*

- *Accounts facility - for ease of keeping track of basic accounts such as petty cash and bank account income and expenditure.*

Hardware

Make sure you buy enough terminals and printers for all positions in your practice, including practice manager, computer operator(s), nurses, doctors, admin/secretary and receptionists. Printers can be shared in some areas, but take care that use does not conflict. Also bear in mind your branch surgeries, even if you do not computerise them straight away.

If the system supplier uses PCs and not just dumb terminals, make sure these are networked and can access several printers around the premises. Also ensure that the PCs are not 'old hat'; you should be thinking about 586 machines as a minimum requirement with a good clock speed of at least 133 mHz or even Pentium processors or 686s. Each should have at least 1 gigabyte hard disk capacity, and if there is one main computer that stores most of your information it should be able to store approximately 2 gigabytes of data, which will allow for future expansion.

With PCs, as well as the specialised GP software there should come some industry-standard software, such as:

- *Windows 95 (or equivalent market leader - MS-DOS).*

- *An integrated package containing a word processor, spreadsheet and database.*

- *Antiviral software would be a good idea.*

Hassle your supplier to try and get as much of this for as little as possible. Compare the prices the supplier quotes with details given in any PC magazine.

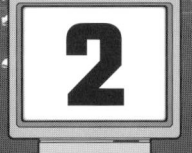

HELP AND ADVICE

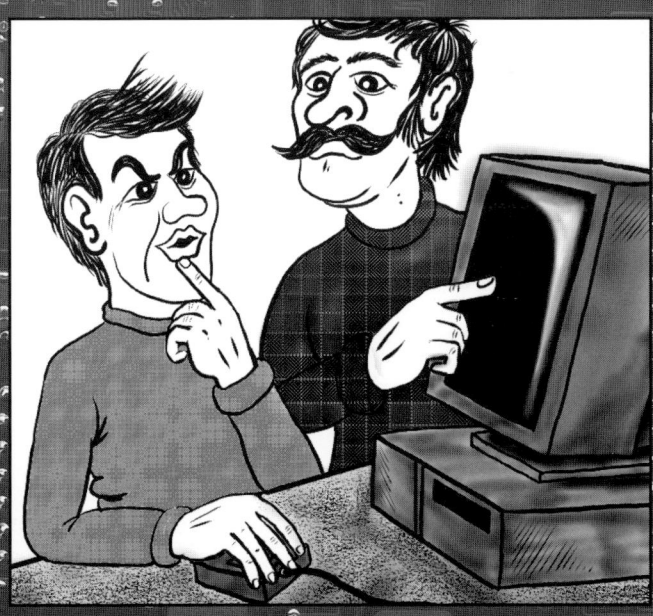

HELP AND ADVICE

There are many people out there who can help you with problems using your computer. Some useful options are given here.

SYSTEM SUPPLIER

You will always have a contract with your supplier for mainte-nance of the hardware, including screens, keyboards, hard disk, processor, printers and modems. They will also provide you with a software maintenance agreement, which guarantees to supply any new versions of the software for your clinical and fundholding sys-tems free of charge.

Your system supplier will provide you with a Helpline number as the first line of enquiry if you have a problem with the operation of your system. (See Section 12 on 'Computer problems').

YOUR HEALTH AUTHORITY AND OTHER SURGERIES

Your Health Authority can supply details of other surgeries who use the same system, and usually these are very willing to help or give you guidance.

THE NATIONAL USER GROUP

Once a supplier has sold a system to you, your details are passed to the National User Group (NUG), which is an independent body formed to liaise between the software supplier and yourselves, the users. You pay a membership fee and are given free help and advice, plus monthly/quarterly newsletters. These keep you up-to-date on further software development and give you access to a strong lob-bying body working on your behalf, who can get bugs fixed and ask for system changes. They also put you in touch with other users in your area, and users arrange meetings for a get together to share common ground or spread ideas.

Anyone can set up a user group in a particular area, if one is not already present, and invite others to attend to discuss ideas on an informal basis.

There is usually an NUG conference annually to allow greater participation from across the country and to appoint new representatives. This gives you direct access to your system supplier for a question and answer session.

3

EFFECTIVE USE OF A COMPUTER

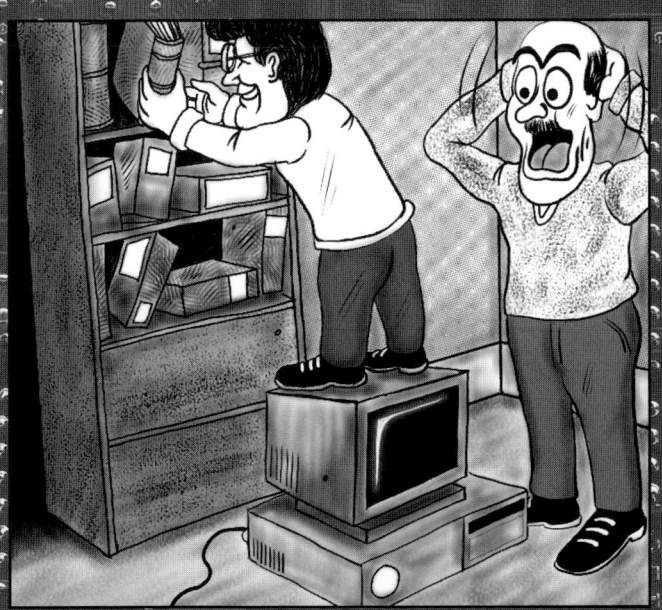

EFFECTIVE USE OF A COMPUTER

This section tries to point the way towards achieving an effective data collection and input system, so that the information is up-to-date, easily accessible and, above all, correct.

A NEW COMPUTER SYSTEM

Obviously, the first step is to have on your system an up-to-date list of all patients registered with your doctors, for all Health Authority areas you may cover. To achieve this, liaise with each relevant Health Authority and agree a paper version of who you both think should be on the list. When this has been corrected and agreed, you should be able to download a version of your list from each Health Authority directly onto your computer via tape cartridge or diskettes. If you need to, you can get help and advice from your computer supplier at this stage.

This will give you your basic information - the age/sex register.

PAPERFLOW

Your next task will be to ensure that the details on paper get to the right person for entry onto the computer system without bypassing any crucial stage.

It would be ideal to rubber stamp all paperwork with a 'C' for 'computer', the absence of which warns anyone handling it, that it has not been through the appropriate channels first.

For a short period of time it would be worthwhile checking all paperwork being sent to the Health Authority or being filed. Ensure that the details required are on the computer already, and that none have bypassed the chain. Once you are happy that nothing is being missed, you can dispense with this procedure.

This sort of exercise could be undertaken for each discrete area of data entry, such as:

- *New registrations - to keep the list up-to-date.*
- *New patient registration exams - to keep health promotion on target.*
- *Repeat prescriptions - for drug updates, issues and reviews.*
- *Change of name, address, etc.*
- *Receipt of notes and returns.*
- *Cervical cytology results - for review dates, recall and targets.*
- *Child immunisation entry - for recall and targets.*
- *Tetanus and travel immunisations - for patient information.*
- *Summary information - updated from incoming mail.*

Do not rush into doing too much too soon. Learn one part of the system thoroughly, then move on to the next.

STAFF TRAINING AND ALLOCATION

Identify who is going to enter each section of information onto the computer and ensure that they receive plenty of training. They must understand the main procedures needed to operate the computer and enter data correctly.

System suppliers should provide some training sessions in the price of buying their system; insist on this if you can. Do not agree to learn too much in one session; get them to train on different days, so that the information sinks in and you have a chance to use the previous training.

Is there someone at the surgery who could be involved in ALL the training sessions and who could become your 'guru'? This would be useful for continuity of information, and they could supplement and enforce the supplier training sessions at a later stage.

Apart from supplier training, perhaps you could visit a surgery in your area that uses the same system to exchange ideas and pick up useful hints and tips.

If you are using a PC-based system with some industry-standard software, it's worth considering college courses that usually run for one term. They provide a basic introduction to most PC packages, including Windows, spreadsheets and word processing.

Remember the famous computing expression -

GIGO - Garbage In, Garbage Out

Allow staff the necessary time to enter the required data, as too short a time will lead to a rushed job, which might be inaccurate. Aim to have them enter at a 'quiet' time, as interruptions are often also to blame for mistakes.

REQUIRED INFORMATION

You need to decide what is going to be recorded on computer. Can you identify exactly which items of information you need to store for future reference?

This is a difficult area as there is a lot of information floating about in a surgery. As a rough guide, enter the minimum amount of data to satisfy the sections already outlined on the previous page **plus** these requirements:

- *your health promotion programmes,*
- *specialist clinics,*
- *item-of-service claims for checking payments.*

Spend a short time working out what the useful information is from your existing manual/clerical procedures - it will be of benefit in the long run. From experience, I have seen masses of data being entered, a large proportion of which is redundant.

Once you have decided on what should be entered, decide **how** to enter it. There may be various ways of inputting the data onto computer, but one standard method should be used by everyone. This applies to those who enter the item, but more importantly to those who need to know how it was entered, in order to access necessary information easily.

This brings into play two more important fundamentals to good computing practices - see 'Documentation' (p42) and 'Read codes' (Section 6).

4

COMPUTERISATION OF CARD-BASED SYSTEMS

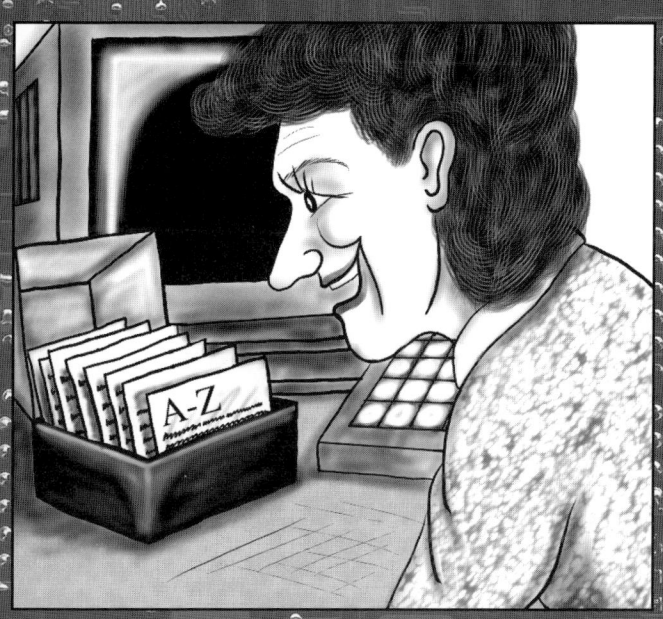

COMPUTERISATION OF CARD-BASED SYSTEMS

Card-based index systems work quite well for the recall of patients for clinics such as hypertension, diabetes, cytology, family planning, etc. However, this takes intensive effort to produce the recalls and to maintain the information. Therefore, these index systems are ideal for entry onto computer.

Patients' summary cards are also ideal fodder for direct entry onto computer, to build up the clinical data gradually.

RECALL SYSTEMS

Most computer systems have the ability to store dates against specific Read codes (see Section 6) for recall purposes, and, together with a good facility for searching these dates, provide the basis for a really good computerised recall system. They also provide basic search facilities that create groups of patients with similar criteria, thus enabling standard letters to be printed for a particular group.

Below are a few pointers to achieving these objectives.

- Identify the important details from the index card and find an equivalent code on your system. Work through all the cards systematically entering the same type of information.

- Make sure that the information on the cards is factually correct - this may involve looking up the clinical notes also. Do not assume that you have all the patients in your index system; do a bit of checking on patients who may be in similar groups. ☞

- Once you have entered details correctly onto computer, ensure you have a system in place to keep the records up-to-date. Write some simple instructions for those people involved in this process.

- Set up a regular searching exercise to identify the patients to be recalled, say on a monthly basis. Print the lists and store them for reference for a year, so that you have a record that the letter has been sent (or allow the system to record this fact in the patient's computerised record, if that is possible on your system).

- Create a standard letter that can be printed regularly for all patients who have been found in the monthly search. This allows individual details to be substituted at the time of printing and is called a 'mailmerge' facility. Your system should have it.

- A little effort in formatting the address information precisely can greatly reduce the work of stuffing envelopes if window types are used. It's easy to print two small dots either side of the page where it needs to be folded.

- It is worth considering using FREEPOST envelopes if you require responses from your patients when you recall them. That way you will increase the response and also identify errors in your data that can be rectified.

SUMMARY CARDS

Patients' summary cards can also be worked through in a similar fashion, but great care should be exercised over who enters the data, whether they are medically qualified and who is finally responsible. Our practice has a policy that clerical staff can enter the data, but if there is a query about the appropriate Read code to be used, it gets passed to a GP or nurse for verification first.

Start at the beginning of the alphabet and work through the records methodically, using a list to highlight any notes that could not be found at the time.

Keep the system up-to-date by introducing a system where the GPs themselves enter more summary details directly onto computer, or get the GP to highlight problems on incoming mail, which can then be transferred onto computer by clerical staff.

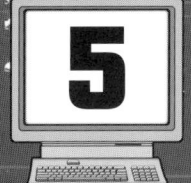

COMPUTERISATION OF AN APPOINTMENT SYSTEM

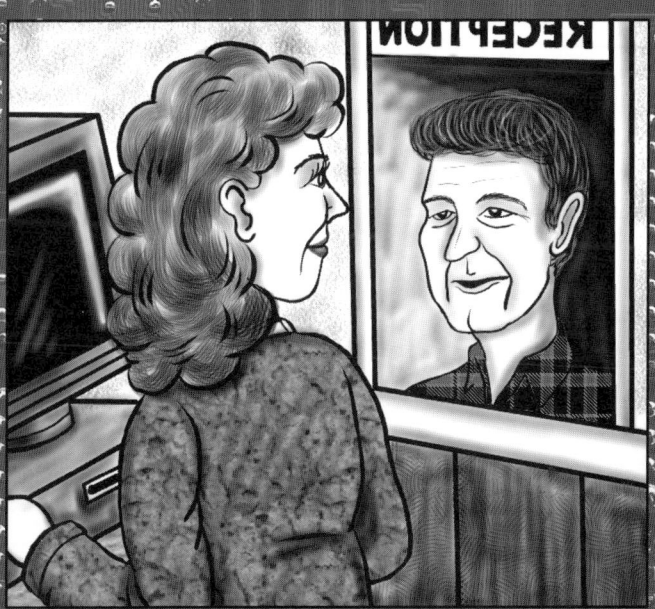

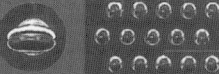

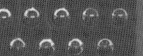
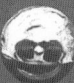

COMPUTERISATION OF AN APPOINTMENT SYSTEM

This section gives some step-by-step ideas for the implementation of a fully computerised appointment system, and works on the assumption that you are already using your computer for the basic patient registration details.

TRAINING

This is probably the most important aspect of starting up a successful appointment system. All staff at your surgery probably make appointments of varying kinds throughout their day's work. Investigate the possibility of getting the staff together for a thorough training session with your software supplier's trainer. If this is not possible, assess whether there is someone who could be trained individually with the view to passing on their knowledge to the rest in small groups.

DUMMY APPOINTMENT SESSIONS

Set up some practice sessions, so that everyone can have a go at making appointments to improve their confidence. This does help when it comes to the crunch and you throw away your books. Listen to ideas that might surface; a lot of pitfalls can be avoided in this way. Set up each session as though it were the real thing - GP sessions for a week, to be carried forward and appointments booked.

At this point, see if someone is willing to be responsible for setting up the sessions on a regular basis for the future rotas.

GRADUAL STEPS

Once you are happy that everyone is familiar with the screens and concepts, begin booking appointments on computer for just two GPs. Although this means remembering which to use, computer or book, as long as you have crossed out the clinics in the book that are to be entered onto computer, you should not go wrong.

Continue like this for a couple of weeks, or until all staff are comfortable with the system, then convert the rest of the GPs. Leave the nurses' and/or outside consultants' sessions for another stage. This spreads the process out a little and allows things to settle gradually, ironing out wrinkles as you go. All of our practice staff were keen to get all appointments computerised, once they had overcome the initial trial period for two GPs.

DOCUMENTATION

I believe that documentation is very important in the effective use of any computerised system. It provides essential information to every user about the way in which items are to be entered to produce standardised data.

Once you have organised the data entry of one particular section of information, write brief, clear instructions on the method of entry, using terms to be seen on screen. It should tell the reader exactly what to press at which point and what is expected of them. Try not to make the instructions too wordy, but at the same time do not miss out any step.

Label each set of instructions clearly and concisely for ease of looking up, and then place them in a folder that is accessible to everyone in the practice. Use this manual to store other pieces of information about the system, especially contact names and numbers, emergency procedures, etc.

Also, provide subsets of the relevant documentation to different groups of staff, depending on their areas of responsibility. Thus nurses can easily identify what they need to do and receptionists can keep their instructions handy on the front desk.

Remember to keep these manuals up-to-date, both when you introduce new procedures and when new NHS strategies require processes to be amended. Then tell everyone about these instructions and the manual - a good way to get everyone working towards the same goals and achieving the same standards of data input.

BENEFITS

It's good to bear in mind the benefits a computerised appointment system might bring. These include:

- *Keeping track of patients who did not keep their appointments.*
- *Finding out a patient's forgotten appointment date and time.*
- *Patient waiting times.*
- *Volume of patients seen by GPs and nurses.*

THE FINAL STAGE

Leading on from complete computerisation of appointments, each GP can access his/her own appointment list for the day, noting how long patients have waited, and assessing who should or could be seen next.

Usually, consultation mode and the appointment list go hand-in-hand, thus ensuring that consultations are created for each patient seen. This will provide more accurate consultation figures for monthly assessment and Annual Report details. Most systems provide automatic figures for any period, broken down into GP/nurse and place of consultation.

6

READ CODES

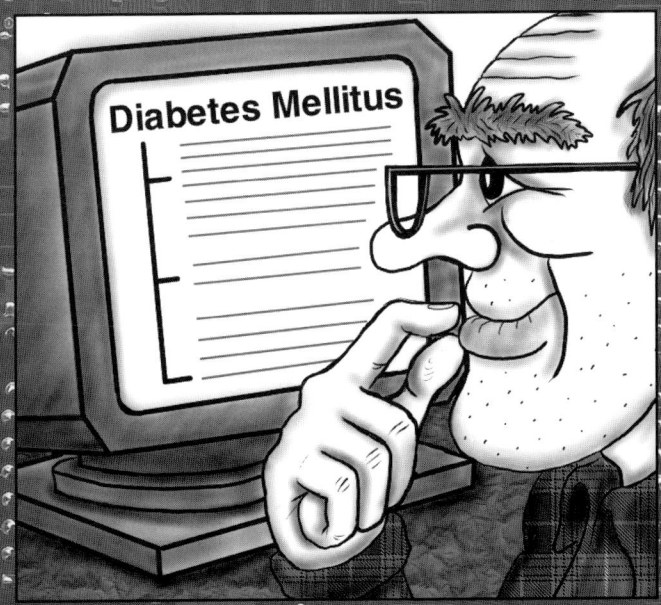

READ CODES

The retrieval and manipulation of data entered onto a computer can be a sizeable problem when you consider all the different ways of expressing the same information. If different terminology is used for a certain disease, then someone conducting an end-of-year search on the computer to identify this disease group will come across initial problems:

- *What do we tell the computer to search for?*
- *What if there were typing mistakes?*
- *What if a certain GP placed this disease under an entirely different category?*

All GP computer systems now adhere to a standard set of codes for any clinically-related information, called Read codes, named after Dr James Read who first introduced the idea. These codes have a structure called a 'hierarchy', which determines to which category of illness or operation they belong. When you are entering data using words, only the Read code linked to that description is stored on computer.

It would be handy if all staff entering clinical data were to have access to a list of the highest code groups, which start with either a number from 0-9 or a letter from A-Z. This helps them to identify the condition being entered and to which category it belongs, so that it is correctly linked as a diagnosis or an operation (see Table 1).

Table 1 - Read code chapters

Chapter	Chapter name
0	Occupations
1	History/symptoms
2	Examinations/signs
3	Diagnostic procedures
4	Laboratory procedures
5	Radiology/physics in medicine
6	Preventive procedures
7	Operations, procedures, sites
8	Other therapeutic procedures
9	Administration
A	Infectious/parasitic diseases
B	Neoplasms
C	Endocrine/nutritional/metabolic/ immunological diseases
D	Blood/blood forming organs diseases
E	Mental disorders
F	Nervous system/sense organ diseases
G	Circulatory system diseases
H	Respiratory system diseases

J	Digestive system diseases
K	Genitourinary system diseases
L	Pregnancy/childbirth
M	Skin/subcutaneous tissue diseases
N	Musculoskeletal/connective tissue disorders
P	Congenital anomalies
Q	Perinatal conditions
R	[D] Symptoms, signs, ill-defined conditions
S	Injury and poisoning
T	Causes of injury/poisoning

The following is an example of the hierarchy of Read codes:

As you can see from the Read code chapters in Table 1, selecting the Full Classification and then C for 'Endocrine/nutritional/metabolic/immunological diseases', gives you the following list:

Endocr/nutr/metab/immun. disease .... C....

Disorders of thyroid gland .... C0...

Other endocrine gland diseases .... C1...

Nutritional deficiencies .... C2...

Other metabolic and immunity disorders .... C3...

Endocrine, nutritional, metabolic or immunity disorders OS .... Cy...

Endocrine, nutritional, metabolic or immunity disorder NOS .... Cz...

Selecting 'Other endocrine gland disease' (C1), gives the next sub-division:

Other endocrine gland disease .... **C1**...

Diabetes mellitus .... **C10**..

Other disorders of pancreatic internal
secretion .... **C11**..

Parathyroid gland disorders .... **C12**..

Disorders of pituitary gland and its
hypothalamic control .... **C13**..

Diseases of thymus gland .... **C14**..

Disorders of adrenal glands .... **C15**..

Ovarian dysfunction .... **C16**..

Testicular dysfunction .... **C17**..

Polyglandular dysfunction and related
disorders .... **C18**..

Other and unspecified endocrine disorders .... **C1z**..

Selecting 'Diabetes mellitus' (C10) gives the following lower subdivision:

Diabetes mellitus .... **C10**..

Diabetes mellitus with no mention of
complication .... **C100**.

Diabetes mellitus with ketoacidosis .... **C101**.

Diabetes mellitus with hyperosmolar coma .... **C102**.

Diabetes mellitus with ketoacidotic coma .... **C103**.

Diabetes mellitus with renal manifestation .... **C104**.

Diabetes mellitus with ophthalmic
manifestation .... **C105**.

Diabetes mellitus with neurological
manifestation .... **C106**.

Diabetes mellitus with peripheral circulatory
disorder .... **C107**.

Diabetes mellitus with other specified manifestation ....*C10y.*

*Diabetes mellitus with unspecified complication.**C10z.*

Selecting 'Diabetes mellitus with renal manifestation' gives the final subdivision:

Diabetes mell. with nephropathy ....*C104.*

Diabetes mellitus, juvenile type, with renal manifestation...*C1040*

Diabetes mellitus, adult onset, with renal manifestation...*C1041*

Diabetes mellitus NOS with renal manifestation *C104z*

As you can see, wherever there is a following full stop, there is a lower level of description that can be selected.

To enter the final diagnosis of 'Diabetes mellitus with hyperosmolar coma' just type DIAB MELL and you will be shown the lower level list from which to choose, thus avoiding working your way down the list from the very top.

Even simpler, if you know the code for your required entry, just type that, i.e. C102.

Whenever you search for 'Diabetes mellitus' (C10), you will always find everyone who has been entered as 'Diabetes mellitus with ketoacidosis' (C101) AND everyone who has been entered as 'Diabetes mellitus, adult onset, with renal manifestation' (C1041).

WARNING

There are times when you must pay attention to which selection you make from the lists given, as you may enter the wrong description in the wrong section of the Read codes. The following is an example:

You enter COUGH to identify the correct code, and the following list is displayed:

Whooping cough **A33**

Cough **171**

Pertussis vaccination **655**

Psychogenic cough **E2611**

Pneumonia with whooping cough **H243**

Smokers' cough **H3101**

[D]Cough **R062**

(This is just a sample of the full list displayed).

If you refer back to Table 1, you can see that A33 is grouped under 'Infectious/parasitic disease', 171 is just 'History/symptoms', 655 is a 'Preventive procedure', E2611 is classed as a 'Mental disorder', and so on. Thus you could quite easily record that a patient has a respiratory system disease (using H3101) when in fact it is just a symptom with no other clinical implication. You have been warned!

See APPENDIX A for details of the leaflet *The impact on GP practices* produced by the NHS Executive about Information Management & Technology.

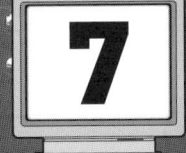

COMPUTER AND
DATA SECURITY

COMPUTER AND DATA SECURITY

Once you have bought your computer system, it is a good idea to carry out a few simple procedures to prevent theft and damage.

First of all, cover all your computer equipment on your insurance policy. You will need to provide all the types, models and serial numbers of every piece of equipment. Keep a list of these somewhere safe and remember to update them if equipment is replaced.

Have a word with your local Crime Prevention Officer who will make recommendations. The following are some worthy considerations:

- *Security marking/tagging - aluminium foil plates with individually etched serial numbers that cannot be dissolved, chipped, peeled or melted off.*

- *Tamper-proof polyester bar-code labels - when removed they leave a checked residue, so tampering can be seen.*

- *Tamper-proof vinyl labels - which break up on attempted removal.*

- *Chrome polyester labels - supplied on continuous stationery, so they can be custom printed and numbered on your own printer.*

- *Stencil - use of a personalised stencil with a compound applied over it, to mark plastic casings permanently.*

- *Fixing - specialised computer locks, which are attached through the casing of the equipment and fixed to an immovable object, such as a desk or wall.*

Nowadays the trend is to steal just the microchips from within the casing of PCs and CPUs. None of the above security devices will stop this, unless your premises are totally secure. However, you do not need to worry too greatly, as usually the only piece of equipment with a chip is the main processor, which you can tuck away somewhere inconspicuously. The terminals and printers around the open office do not contain any chips and are therefore not in danger. PCs are vulnerable, as they do contain their own processing chips, so extra caution is needed in the positioning of these items.

Use of invisible marking systems is all well and good, but it does not tell the potential thief that it has been marked. So put bright stickers on all the equipment to show that it's not worth stealing in the first place. This will be a lot less inconvenient than losing it and having it recovered by the Police at a later date.

Your surgery should already have an alarm system, and making sure it is serviced regularly is vital to the safety of drugs, computers, patients' notes and other equipment held on the premises. With all of the extra electrical wiring and circuitry around, it would be wise to have a qualified electrician check the appliances regularly. This is covered in general health and safety policies.

DATA SECURITY

This is another area that needs careful consideration. Having taken steps to secure the physical hardware, it would be ludicrous not to take reasonable steps to prevent damage or loss to information stored on your computer system.

To this end, each supplier will advise you of activities that should be undertaken regularly to reduce the risk of damage or loss. Below are a few standard precautions that are usually specified.

Backups
This applies equally well to the main clinical/fundholding processor and any PC that you may have on the premises, and should be

carried out every day. It copies data from the main system onto either tape or diskette, to be stored in a safe place overnight. This then provides the most recent set of data in cases where a corruption occurs on your hard disk and the data stored there cannot be accessed.

Arrange for someone to be responsible for taking the tape or diskettes home at night and bringing them back the following day.

Set up a logbook of when the backup is done and by whom, and whether it was successful or not. This helps when problems arise or one person takes over from another.

Set up a cycle of tapes/diskettes, such as 5/6 labelled for each day of the working week. These can be used on the appropriate day and stored safely off-site; or just store the latest off-site.

NB Installations of new versions of software should also be recorded in this logbook and the diskettes also stored safely or off-site.

Validation/integrity check

Some form of validation process will usually be supplied within your clinical software, which should be run on a regular basis, to check that the data being written is correct and linked in the expected fashion. Sometimes odd bits of data may become detached from a patient's record and this option would relink details.

Uninterruptible power supply (UPS)

Your supplier will probably recommend that you have one of these devices installed. Where power fluctuation or failure occurs, the UPS will protect the data by providing a continuing electrical supply until it shuts down the system in a controlled manner. It will then restart the system automatically once the power is returned.

In the event of electrical interference due to a storm, turn off as many pieces of equipment as possible, such as terminals and printers.

This is because the UPS sometimes can act as a conduit for a lightning strike and, whilst protecting the main processor, it diverts the current down the lines to any other equipment that may be attached to the processor.

Parallel/twin systems

This is a method of backup usually used in a totally paperless practice. It relies on a complete duplicate of the main processor and its database being updated simultaneously with the first. If there is corruption on the master or primary system, all processes can be switched to the secondary system. Obviously this is quite costly, but it has been done in some practices.

Off-site backup

You could have an arrangement with a nearby practice to share systems when you encounter hardware problems. This would be possible if you had similar terminals or printers or even PCs, but also if you had the same software and the data could be kept separate. This option would need to be explored with the supplier.

THE *DATA PROTECTION ACT* 1984

Every computerised surgery must be registered under the *Data Protection Act* 1984; it is a criminal offence not to be.

The Act applies to personal data that is in some way processed automatically, i.e. held on computer. It gives the individual certain rights to gain access to the data and check its correctness, whilst also ensuring that those who process the data on computer are open about its use and follow guidelines against illegal use, and accidental or malicious damage.

Personal data	Any information held about a living, identifiable individual.
Data user	Those who control the entry and use of personal data. This can be any company or organisation, both public and private, no matter how small. A data user need not necessarily own a computer; the information may be obtained through an agency, such as a computer bureau.
Data subject	The individual to whom the stored data relates.

How to register

A registration form may be obtained from any Post Office.

You must supply the following information:

- *your surgery's name and address;*
- *details of the personal data to be held;*
- *the purpose for which it is to be used;*
- *the source(s) from which the data is obtained;*
- *the recipients of any such data, i.e. to whom it is shown or passed;*
- *any overseas countries to which the data may be transferred.*

Registration is for an initial period of three years for which there is one fee payable.

Once registered, you must adhere to the details set out above and comply with the EIGHT Data Protection Principles:

❶ *To obtain and process data fairly and lawfully.*

❷ *To hold data only for lawful purposes described in your registration.*

❸ *To disclose data only to those people described in your registration.*

❹ *To hold only adequate, relevant data not excessive to the purpose for which it is held.*

❺ *To keep the data accurate and up-to-date.*

❻ *To hold data no longer than is necessary.*

❼ *To allow access to the individual for correction or erasure.*

❽ *To keep data secure.*

SUBJECT ACCESS RIGHTS

This is the part of the *Data Protection Act* 1984 that allows individuals to see the information held about them on computer by the surgery. They can have the information corrected or deleted as appropriate.

How subject access rights work

The individual must make a written request to the surgery, to be supplied with a copy of any personal data held about them on computer. The surgery may charge up to £10 for each request. This request must be responded to within 40 days, or the individual may complain to the Registrar or obtain a court order. The individual then has the right to have any incorrect or misleading data altered.

An individual is entitled to compensation for any damage or distress suffered as a result of loss, damage, destruction, disclosure or illegal access of the personal data, provided that the damage suffered was after 12th September 1984 and that the data user was negligent in its duties under the principles of the Act.

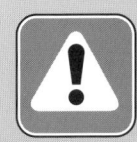 **WARNING!**

The *Data Protection Act* 1984 allows access to anything clinical recorded on computer about the patient from 1984. The *Access to Health Records Act* 1990 only allows the patient to see information about themselves from November 1991. Therefore, be careful in backloading any data about the patient relating to a period between 1984 and 1991 - it should be accurate, but not sensitive.

A series of booklets called the *Data Protection Guidelines* are available free from the Data Protection Office. APPENDIX A provides details of the booklets and the address.

THE *ACCESS TO HEALTH RECORDS ACT* 1990

This Act was established in 1990, but access applies to patient records written from November 1991 onwards. The delay was to allow health professionals to alter their working practices accordingly, i.e. to refrain from writing sensitive comments in the notes that would be to the patient's detriment if seen or heard at that time, but that were relevant to their health care.

As in the *Data Protection Act*, the patient may request access to his/her medical record, or a part of it, and has the right for any inaccurate data to be corrected by the GP. However, if the GP disagrees, the GP may make a note of both sets of details beside the relevant information in the record. A copy of the accessed and/or corrected information is then provided to the patient, if required.

You are required to respond within 40 days from the date of application, if all of the record was written more than 40 days before the application date. Otherwise, where the records were written within this 40-day period, you have 21 days from the date of application to respond.

In certain circumstances, a patient may be represented by another individual for these processes.

8

YOUR COMPUTER AND ITS PERIPHERALS

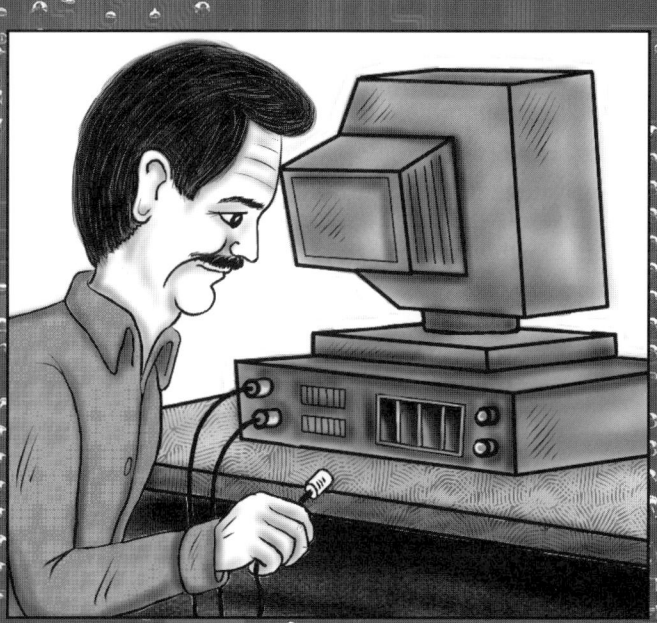

YOUR COMPUTER AND ITS PERIPHERALS

DISK DRIVES

Disk drives are the units in your computer that rotate data storage disks at high speed. There are two main types of disk drive - hard disk drive and floppy disk drive (the common 3½" or the almost redundant 5¼").

Hard disk drive

This is the device inside the main computer, which spins your disk and then allows data to be read or written using a 'head', which floats over the surface picking up the magnetic or electrical signals. This is rather like the operation of a record player - if you can remember those.

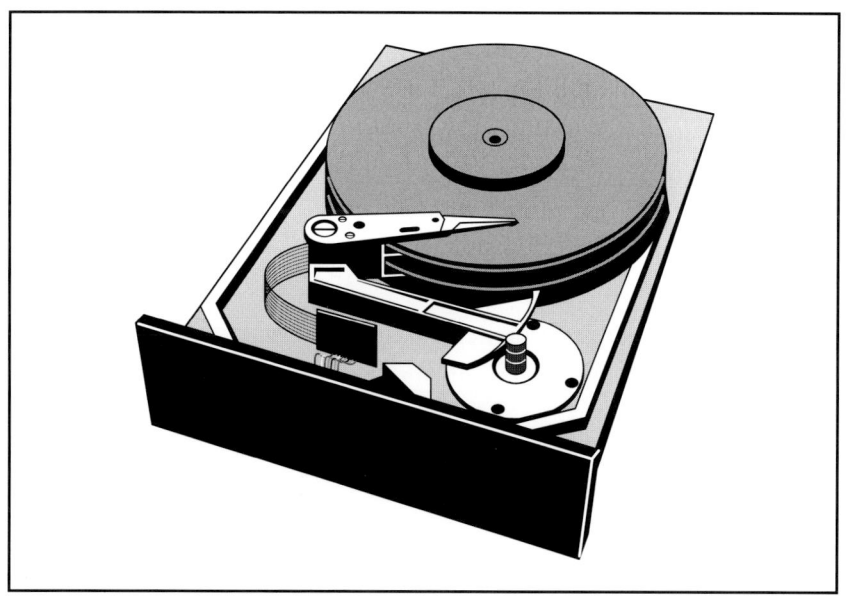

Sometimes data corruption is caused when a power fluctuation occurs, because data was being read or written at the precise moment that the disk slowed from its correct spinning speed. This corruption may be in an area that does not affect the running of the system and is detected and corrected by certain verification procedures run on the system.

Other data corruptions may have a physical cause, in which case it is most apparent and your system will probably not work at all, or make unusual noises. In this case, report it immediately to your Helpline, who will call in an engineer as soon as possible.

Some data corruptions manifest themselves when a backup is carried out. In this instance, the backup will report errors which you should make note of. Sometimes the supplier will recommend that one error on backup is not sufficient to worry about, but that two episodes should be reported immediately.

Floppy disk drive (see opposite)

This is, in principle, the same mechanism as the hard disk drive, but you insert the media to be read or written - the 5¼" or 3½" diskettes.

You would use this drive to copy new versions of software, provided by your supplier, from floppy diskette onto the hard disk. Also you could 'download' information from your clinical or fundholding system onto diskette, say, for use by the Health Authority in GP Links testing, or for incorporation into another software package on a different system.

You may need to format diskettes for the above purpose, although some are supplied ready formatted. Occasionally, diskettes will not format correctly, in which case an error message on screen will tell you so. Use another diskette and put the faulty one aside. Most diskettes have some form of warranty - look carefully at the box for details.

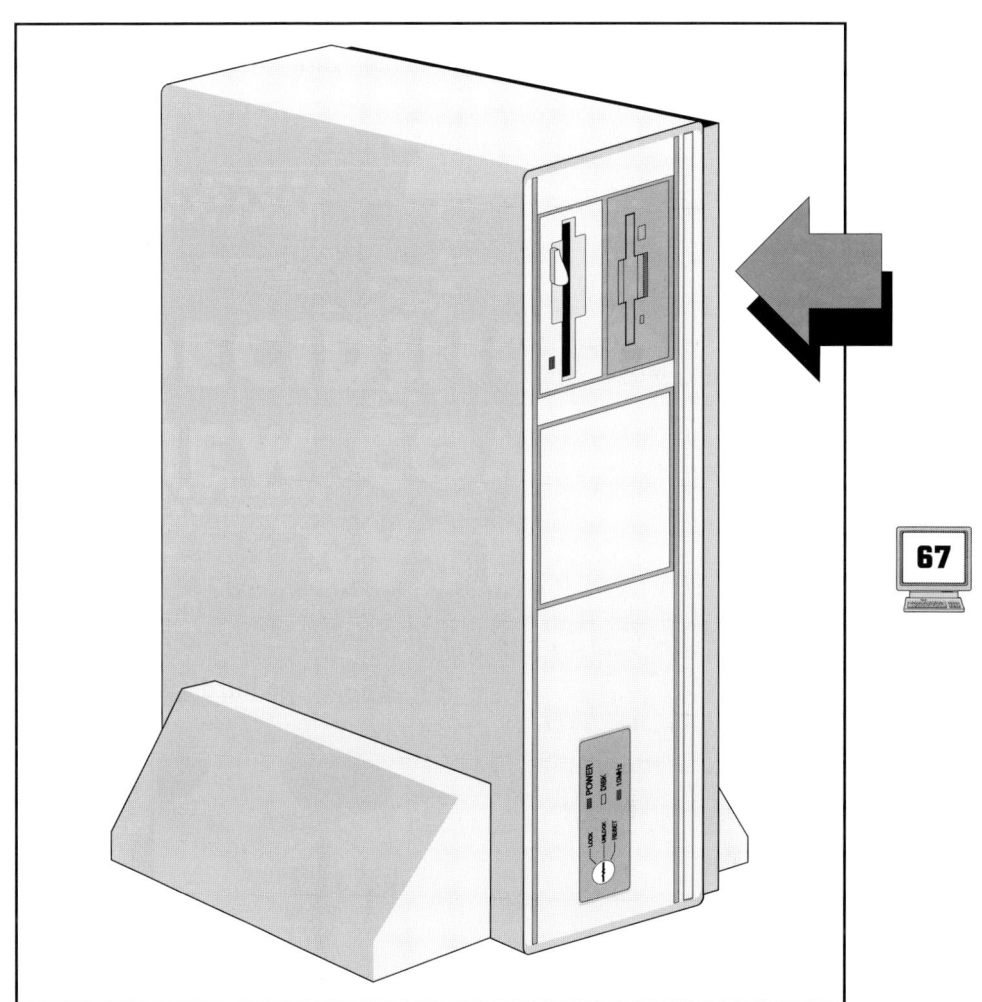

COMPUTER PERIPHERALS

A peripheral is any device connected to your main computer system, other than just a keyboard or screen. Printers, modems and CD-ROMs are all types of peripheral. What follows is a brief description of what they are, what they can do for you and the problems that you might encounter with them.

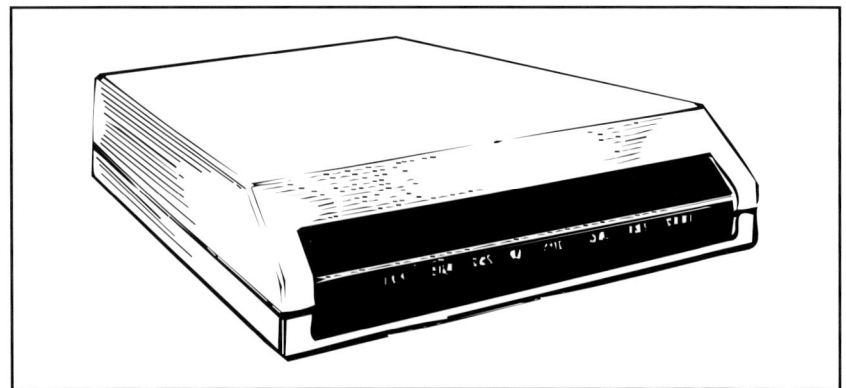

Modem

This stands for 'modulator/demodulator' and is the box that converts computer signals into telephone signals and *vice versa*. There would be one attached at either end of a telephone line before the signal reached the main computer. The modem is physically attached to your computer, but is then plugged into an outgoing telephone line. In our surgery, this outgoing line is where the fax machine is also plugged in. The modem can be plugged in when needed, and in this instance anyone trying to send you a fax will get the engaged tone. All modems must be approved by British Telecom for use on their lines. Those approved adhere to certain strict standards and are the normal type supplied.

You would have the modem connected if you wished to link your system to another system, such as the pathology laboratory for automatic download of test results. It would also be used in any link to the Health Authority computerised system or simply for using terminals and printers at a branch surgery.

Modems quite often lose the signal, in which case there is sometimes a little red button on the back where the wires come out, which can be depressed to reset it.

Your system supplier may use this method to dial up your system in order to correct problems you have reported. It is well worth considering having a totally separate telephone line dedicated for this purpose alone, as remembering to swap from fax to modem is a constant source of aggravation at our practice.

Multiplexor

This is also a box-like device that attaches to your main processor. It allows any peripherals you may have at branches to communicate successfully with the main processor.

The connection order from a branch to the main processor is shown here.

The various electrical signals are sent by the remote peripherals and can be amalgamated and sent to the modem, which converts them to a telephone signal. The open telephone line transmits the signals to the main surgery where they are decoded by the modem then separated by the multiplexors and allowed access to the main computer.

All of this takes a very few seconds to send and receive, while at the same time the signals are verified at both ends so that data is not lost. This verification process also checks to make sure the data is not tampered with in any way, but it is very difficult to say what has actually happened in such cases of data loss/damage.

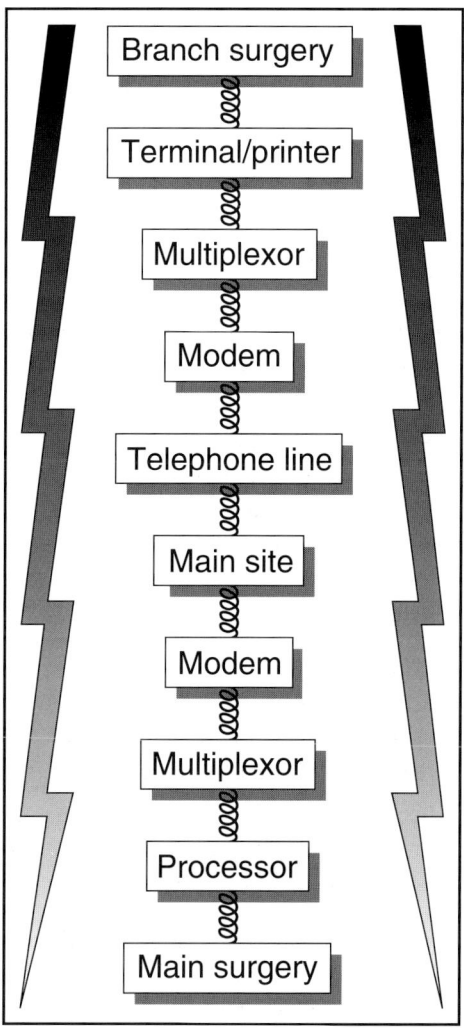

Printers

There are many different types of printers on the market today. They vary in price, quality of printing, variety of typeface, speed, and ability to print on different media and in colour. Your surgery needs to decide what it is you want your printer to achieve.

Secretarial requirements are usually single-sheet feed, with the ability to print in several typefaces, if necessary, and perhaps to feed in envelopes. The quality should be reasonably good for mailing accounts and referrals. An example of a printer capable of this is any type of deskjet or inkjet printer.

Clinical system requirements are usually of a slightly lesser quality - a workhorse, reliable, easy to use and with continuous paper feed. This copes with printing prescriptions, reports and mailshots for recalls. A standard dot-matrix printer will cope with this type of printing.

Fundholding requirements are slightly different again, as wide reports are available. In this case a wide-carriage dot-matrix printer may be an option.

If you intend to use a PC on the system and would like to produce a good quality Annual Report or other graphic presentations, a good quality deskjet or inkjet printer would be a requirement. These can usually print to acetate for use on overhead projectors.

Mouse

This is a device that substitutes for the use of a keyboard in some circumstances. It is a small hand-held device, with two or three buttons, that is rolled around on a mat to manipulate an arrow on the screen. It is used to point to graphic representations (icons) of actions that you wish to undertake by pressing the appropriate button.

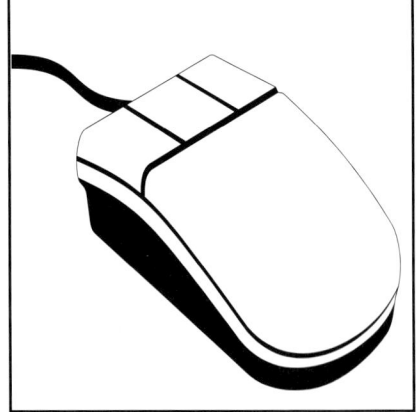

A mouse is most frequently used with PC systems where standard packages, such as Windows, rely on the use of a mouse to select options from a list.

I believe that some clinical systems might have this option in future, but I have not seen one demonstrated so far.

Scanners/optical character readers (OCR)

This is a device that could be attached to your system in future, to record whole documents against a patient's record. Software can be bought that picks up these scanned images, including the written word, and converts them into a computerised document on screen. This can then be manipulated and stored to a database.

A scanner would be of use if your clinical system provided a facility to read this scanned information into a patient's record automatically; this cannot be too far away, as path lab results are also items of information that can be sent to a computer and be assimilated into a patient's record.

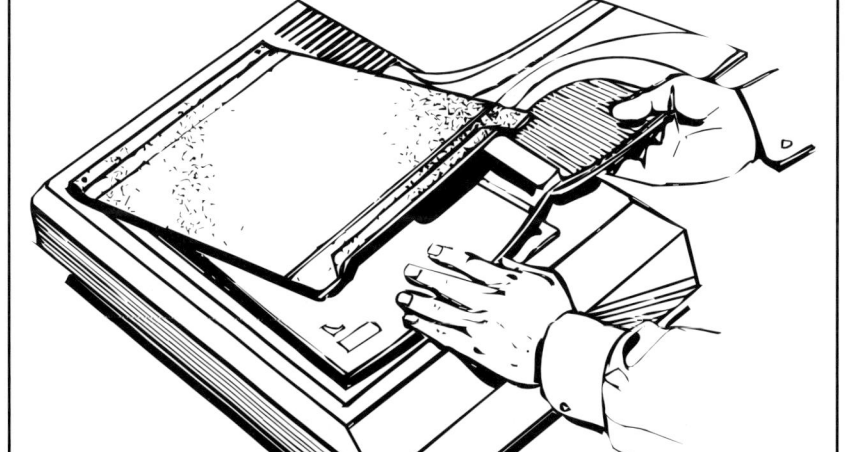

Scanners can record any data, written, printed, graphic or photographed. They can scan coloured images to black and white, or can record to colour if your software and system allows.

The OCR machine was the forerunner of a scanner and is not used so much. It can read only printed data and is very much inferior in quality to the scanners in the shops today.

CD-ROM

This stands for Compact Disk - Read-Only Memory. It is a digital recording of information that can be read by a 'head' and is the same technology used by musical CDs. Drives that read this type of information can be attached to your system, again provided you have the software and your system allows integration.

The type of information available on CD-ROM is now very varied and includes Bodyworks - a medical information system, with moving images. Many medical reference texts are now available on CD-ROM, such as the British National Formulary and certain HMSO publications.

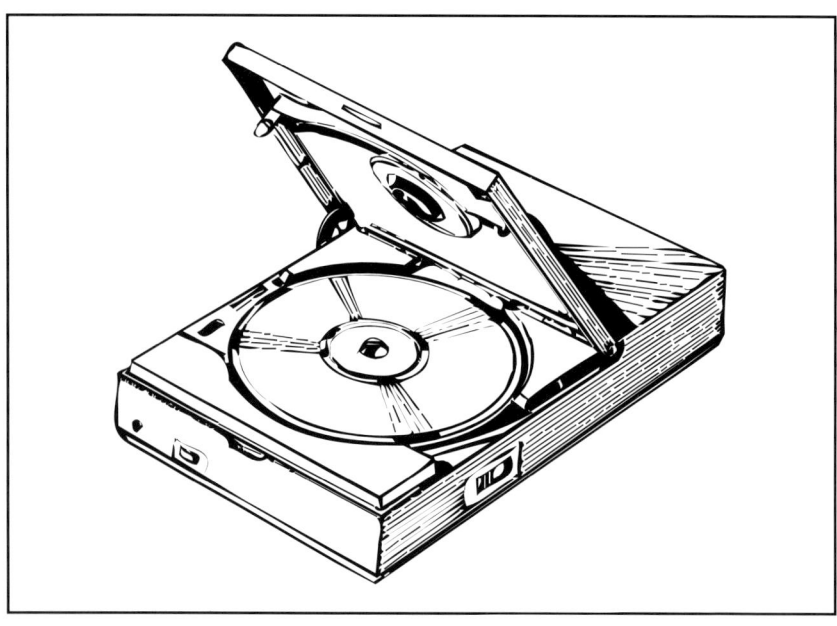

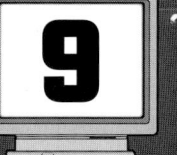

BRITISH
TELCOM LINES

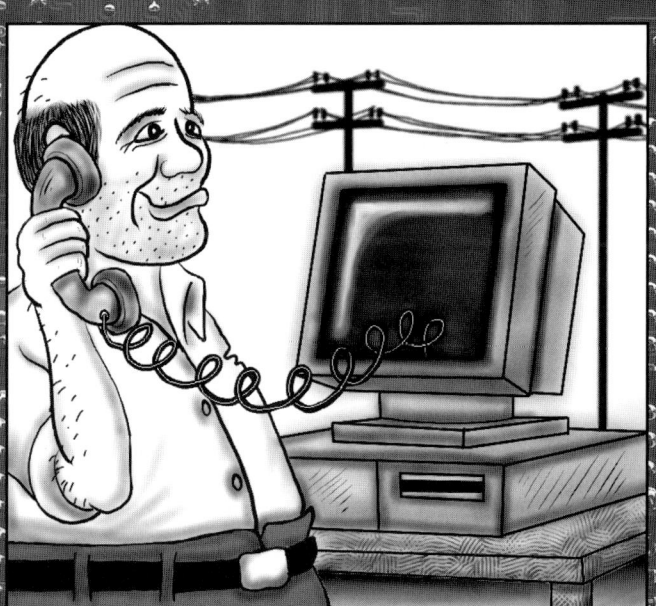

BRITISH TELECOM LINES

There are two alternative methods of connecting your computer to another system - 'dial-up line' and 'land line'.

Dial-up is used where the link is not 'permanent'. The Health Authority uses this method as they dial into many different systems throughout your region. The same applies to your system supplier, who may use this method to solve problems on your system. These link-ups are often of short duration and are probably cost-effective if not too long.

The land line option is more suitable for use over an extended time period, where dial-up as a standard telephone call would not be cheap. This method is often used for connecting to branch surgeries.

When connecting any computer to a telephone line, it is worth considering the following questions:

TELEPHONE LINE CHECKLIST

☐ *Do you require a separate line for this purpose?*

- *YES if the supplier uses this method to dial into your computer to fix faults.*

- *YES if you wish in future to link to the Health Authority or path lab.*

- *YES if you thought of doubling up on your fax line, but this is used frequently and especially overnight.*

☐ *Should you use a standard dial-up line or a land line?*

- *Try to estimate the costs of the standard call charges for a dial-up line - just like making phones calls. Be aware of how long transmissions might take and take account of a branch site where the same method will be used whilst surgeries last.*

- *Land lines necessitate an initial higher installation cost, but the communication line is always open and there is only a maintenance charge, no call charges.*

You must decide which is of benefit to you.

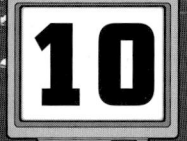

GP/HEALTH AUTHORITY LINKS

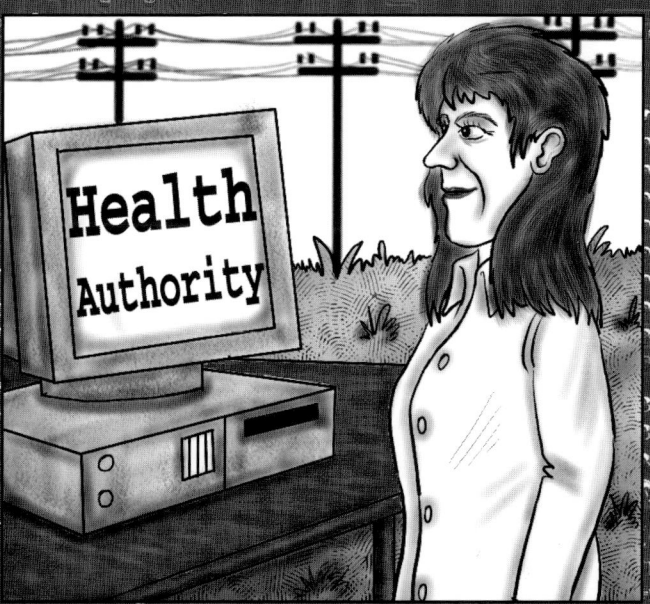

GP/HEALTH AUTHORITY LINKS

WHAT IS 'LINKS'?

This is the process by which surgeries can communicate directly with their Health Authority, via a modem and the telephone line. There are two stages: 'registrations' and then 'items-of-service'. Below are some brief outlines on how to achieve this link and what daily procedures are involved, highlighting benefits along the way.

This allows your Health Authority to receive new registration details directly from your computer on a daily basis and, likewise, allows you to receive updated information about the patient from the Health Authority, such as the NHS number. This was an advantage when the new NHS numbers were allocated automatically.

Table 2 (overleaf) details some of the systems that provide the necessary programs for Links.

THE ROAD TO LINKS

Your computer system should allow you to link to your Health Authority as this is one of the accreditation criteria. Check with your software supplier that you have an up-to-date version of the software with this ability. The box on page 81 is a short guide to the tasks you will need to achieve to link to your Health Authority for registrations transfer.

In our surgery we then ran a parallel system, which entailed entering the registration details on computer **and** still getting all of the GMS1s or medical cards signed by the patient and GP.

Table 2 - Software versions for GP Links

Supplier	System	Version
AAH Meditel	System 5	5.6.4
Ambridge Business Systems Ltd	GP Manager	2.1
Brandt Computer Systems Ltd	Medico	2.0
Egton Medical Information Systems	EMIS	4.3
Exeter GP Systems	Exeter GP Systems	10.0
Hollowbrook Computer Services Ltd.	Micro-Doc	7.1
M-TEC Computer Services (UK)	System HMC	6.0
Medical Care Systems Ltd.	MCS System 7 MCS Medusa MCS 2000	1.0 3.0 2.3
Micro Solutions Ltd.	Surgery Manager	1.0
Microtest Ltd.	Practice Manager (II)	1.0
Seetec Ltd	GP Professional	2.2
Toloui Associates	Geminus	1.0
VAMP Health Ltd.	VAMP Medical Systems VAMP Vision	5.0 1.1

Details accurate as of May '96

- Contact your Health Authority to begin the process. They can give you an implementation plan and target dates for each step. Liaise with them frequently to check progress as timing is quite important.

- Contact your software supplier, to put them in the picture, and they can help you with setting up the system.

- Install a modem and telephone line, if you do not already have one available - check with your supplier. This will also involve setting up a mailbox facility which is hired from either Racal or BT. Again your supplier and the Health Authority will advise you.

- Check your list of present patients with that of the Health Authority. This may take several comparisons, which can be run on your system. Speak to your Health Authority constantly about disagreements. Usually it boils down to your computer being more accurate than theirs. They will usually agree with you over minor details, but will insist on you re-registering patients that they do not have on their list.

- Agree dates for all of these actions and keep the Health Authority informed.

- Once lists are agreed, the Health Authority will set a 'live' date on which they will descend on your practice to test the link using dummy data, followed by the real thing.

- At the same time, you will receive basic training from the Health Authority staff on what it is necessary to do and when. Make notes and get hold of any documentation your software company can provide.

HOW DO THINGS CHANGE AFTER IMPLEMENTATION?

We set up our computer to send and receive data from the mailbox overnight. Hence, first thing in the morning the data can be collected and assimilated into your system. Thus patient records are automatically updated with acceptance details, but you must accept amendments to addresses and NHS numbers individually. Also, you can print details of patients whose notes have been requested for return, so that you can retrieve them from your filing in alphabetical order on a daily basis.

Any changes of detail, such as surname, address, etc., are automatically stored for sending to the Health Authority overnight. This means that the two computer systems always carry identical information of patient details and whereabouts of notes; a great benefit when chasing queries.

At the end of each quarter your computer will be able to provide accurate patient list sizes which the Health Authority will accept without question - an additional benefit. However, do wait until your Health Authority prompts you to run this facility as timing is once again crucial to an exact match of figures.

After your 'parallel run', GMS1s and medical cards do NOT require a GP signature - a great saving in legwork at our practice. These GMS1s and medical cards need only be sent to the Health Authority once every quarter for verification. Thus the forms do not 'go missing' and the patient is already accepted onto the system.

11

COMPUTER CONSUMABLES

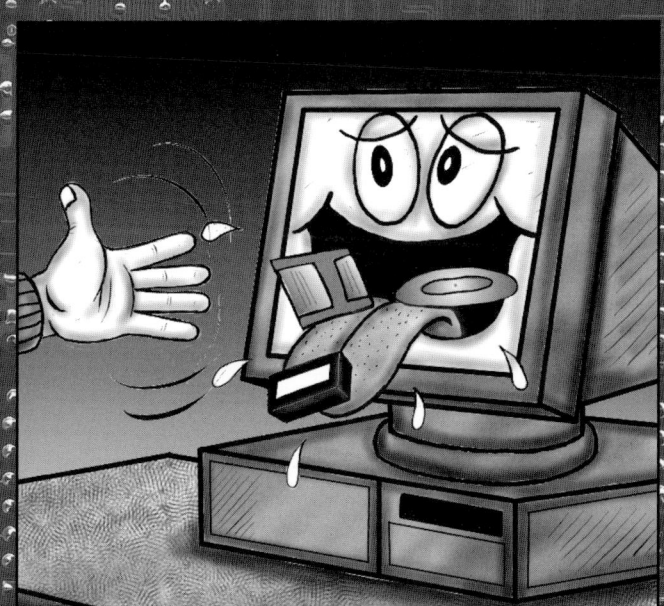

COMPUTER CONSUMABLES

WHAT ARE THEY?

Consumables are the items that are used up daily by running your system, such as paper, diskettes, tapes and print ribbons or cartridges.

WHERE TO LOOK

You can quite often find most of these items at a local computer store, like PC World or Tempo, or a local office supplies shop. You could also buy any substantial computer magazine from your newsagent and look through the hundreds of suppliers - you might find a good deal that's local.

WHICH TYPE?

Make sure you know exactly which type of consumable you require to replace the existing stock by making a note of any serial numbers or details on the packaging. Most handbooks for printers will supply you with the information about ribbons or cartridges. Many people using some form of printer cartridge do look into re-inking. We tried this at my practice and found it to be messy, time-consuming and, in the end, not much cheaper.

Your main computer and any linked PCs will nowadays take either of two standard types of diskette (see Figure 2).

1. *5¼" double-sided high density (which can be already formatted for use) - most PC manufacturers do not build their machines for this type of diskette.*

2. *3½" double-sided high density.*

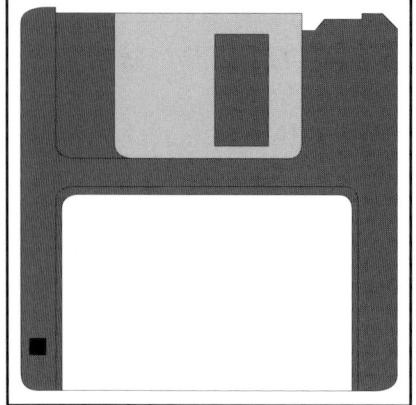 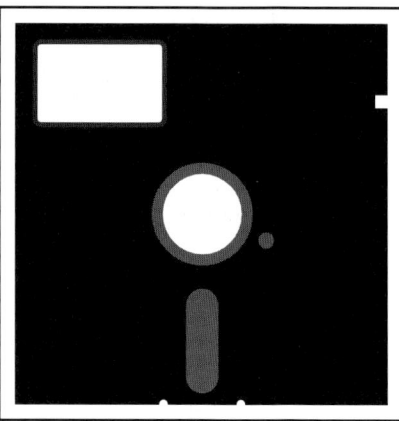

Figure 2
Left: 3½"
floppy
Right: 5¼"
floppy

There are 10 to a box, when prices are quoted. A minimum of three boxes would probably be adequate to make one backup of a PC supplied with software packages.

Diskettes are normally only used to download data from a system to transfer to another unlinked system, e.g. when preparing for Health Authority links, or possibly for keeping a backup of any PC packages that you might buy independently.

Your main system backup is probably done using tape cartridge, which is capable of holding much more information (usually around 120 megabytes compared to the average two megabytes of a 3½" disk) and carries out this operation much more speedily. Your supplier will provide enough of these to begin with, and if they do not, ask.

Printer paper can be bought from any office supplies shop. Hunt around and you might get a preferential rate. Try your local council offices, who have their own internal supplies catalogue at discounted rates that you might be able to use. Also try contacting your local hospital computer department, other local surgeries that are computerised and your Health Authority, who might be persuaded to supply you via your weekly deliveries.

Paper can be of the following types:

- *FANFOLD AND MICROPERFORATED - this is continuous sheets fed automatically using sprocket holes at the side, which are then separated by perforations at the bottom and the sprocket holes discarded at the sides.*
- *SINGLE SHEET - fed in individually, rather like a typewriter, from a paper feed tray attached to the printer.*

Paper size can vary; usually you would require paper with sprocket holes that would reduce to a standard A4 size (29.7 cm x 21 cm). Certain single sheet feed printers can use ordinary photocopier paper, but higher quality or standard headed paper for letters might be required.

For those of you who may be, or are, changing to fundholding, wider paper with ruled lines for complicated reports might be useful. This is called 'music ruled'. Check that one of your printers can take this size.

12

COMPUTER PROBLEMS

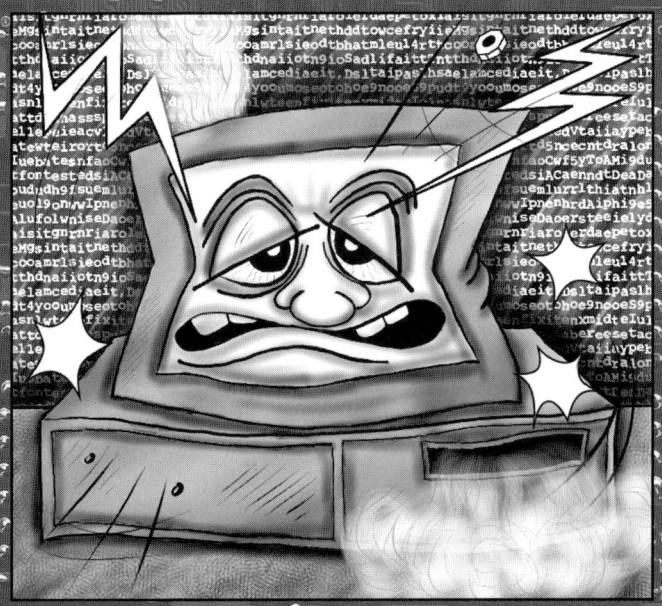

COMPUTER PROBLEMS

Your supplier will have given you a contact number when the system was installed. This gives you access to someone who can sort out any problems you may have, if not directly, then by referring the problem on. This line is usually available 9am to 5pm weekdays and possibly Saturday mornings.

As soon as you experience a problem with the computer system, write down exactly what you were doing at the moment it happened, especially any patient number involved, and whether anyone else was using the system at that time. List any error messages that appeared on the screen. It may be advisable to record them on a 'computer fault report form' and to store these in a file so that any consistent problems with the computer, the software or the user can be identified and dealt with.

If the supplier uses a modem as the support line, make sure it is plugged in before ringing the Helpline. Be ready to quote your reference number or lead partner's name and tell them precisely what has occurred; they need all the pertinent information to be able to solve the fault.

Once you are speaking to the person who will fix your problem, get their name, as you may need to contact them again about this particular problem. Write an account of the problem on the 'computer fault report form' with its eventual resolution, keeping details of dates, if it spreads over a number of days, and any contact names. This will be useful, especially if you have a number of faults with a particular piece of hardware, as this strengthens your case for having it replaced.

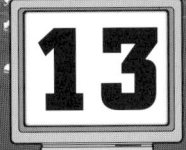

USERS'
WELFARE

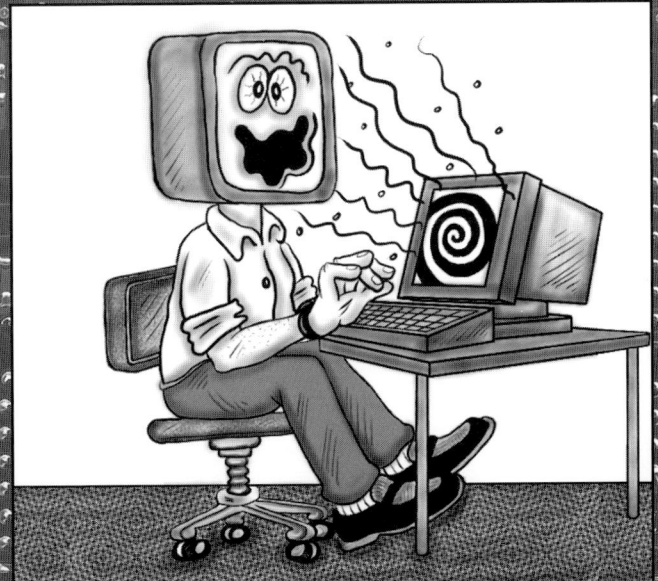

USERS' WELFARE

It is very important that anyone using a screen/VDU and keyboard for a significant part of the working day should be safeguarded against fatigue and strain. There are a number of precautions that can be taken to minimise any untoward effects. The minimum requirements are laid down by the *Health and Safety (Display Screen Equipment) Regulations* 1992.

The chief recommendations of these regulations can be summarised briefly as:

- *Analyse, assess and reduce any risks from the terminals.*
- *Allow regular breaks or change of activity in the work.*
- *Arrange eye tests for employees.*
- *Provide health and safety training.*
- *Provide information about all of the above to the employee.*

There is no evidence to suggest that emissions from screens cause any illness or injury; however, eye tests may well reveal any existing problem. Ensure that glare is cut down and that brightness controls are available on all screens. It may be necessary or more comfortable to the individual to have an anti-glare filter fitted over the screen - these can be bought quite cheaply.

The position one sits at while working at a screen is also very important. The screen should be easily seen without excessive movement of the head up or down. The seated position should be upright, with space for the hands and wrists to rest comfortably on the desk. Maybe an attachment to the side of the screen for copy typing documents could be provided and keyboard extenders for wrists are available.

Appendix A gives details of the leaflet *Working with VDUs*, which summarises the Regulations.

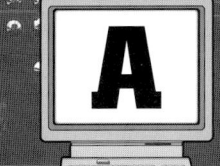

APPENDIX

APPENDIX A

The Data Protection booklets are:

- *Introduction to the Act*
- *The Definitions*
- *The Register and Registration*
- *The Data Protection Principles*
- *Individuals' Rights*
- *The Exemptions*
- *Enforcement and Appeals*
- *Summary for Computer Bureaux*
- *Individuals' Rights Leaflet - 'If there's a mistake on computer about you'*
- *What is Data Protection?*
- *Index of Guidance Notes*
- *Small Business Information pack*
- *Professional Advisers' pack*
- *Student pack*
- *Registration pack*

The address to write to obtain the booklets and gain advice is:

The Office of the Data Protection Registrar
Wycliffe House
Water Lane
Wilmslow
Cheshire SK9 5AF

The Health and Safety Leaflet Working with VDUs can be obtained by mail order from:

HSE Books
PO Box 1999
Sudbury
Suffolk CO10 6FS
Tel: 01787 81165
Fax: 01787 313995

Or from Dillons Bookstores

The Impact on GP Practices: Implementing the infrastructure for Information Management & Technology in the NHS is issued by the Information Management Group of the NHS Executive. For further information contact:

The NHS Executive Headquarters
Department of Health
Quarry House
Quarry Hill
Leeds LS2 7UE
Tel: 01132 545000

B

APPENDIX

APPENDIX B

OTHER READING MATERIAL:

Collins Reference - *Dictionary of computing*

Oftel - *A basic guide to data communications*

NHS Executive - *The impact on GP practices*

The *Access to Health Records Act* 1990 (available as reference in libraries)

The Read codes - a user guide for general practitioners

Computers Aided Medical Systems Ltd (CAMX)

Tannery Buildings

Woodgate

Loughborough

Leicestershire LE11 2TQ

The following publications also offer sections on computing:

Pritchard P, Low K, Whalen M. *Management in general practice.* Oxford: Oxford General Practice Series 8.

Dean J. *Making sense of practice finance.* Oxford: Radcliffe Medical Press.

Preece J. *The use of computers in general practice.* London: Churchill Livingstone.

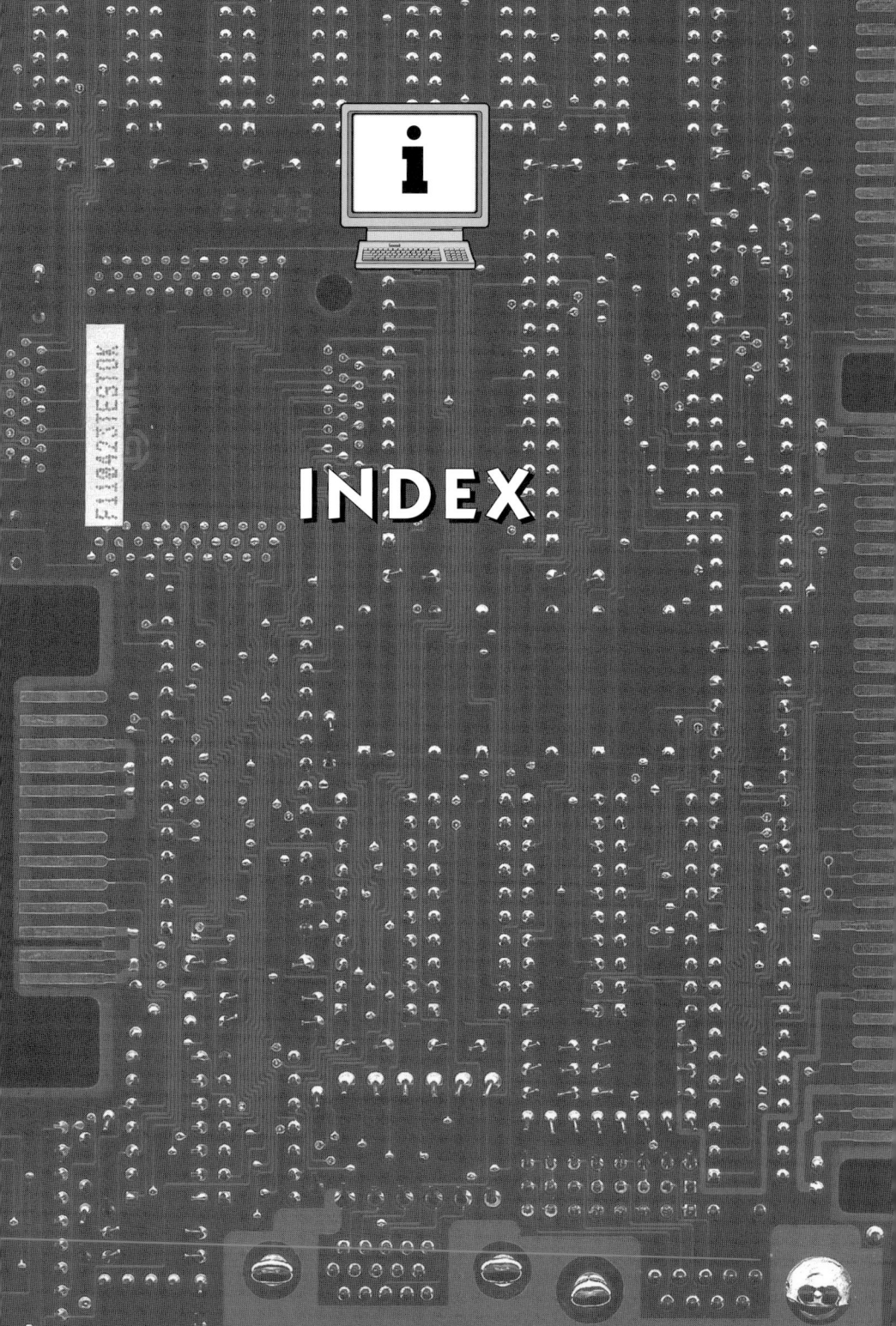

INDEX

107

T

U

109

V

W